# RECIPES 4
## R A W   F O O D

A COLLECTION OF **20**
AWESOME RAW SOUP
RECIPES THAT ARE EASY,
FUN, HEALTHY, AND
NUTRITIOUS.

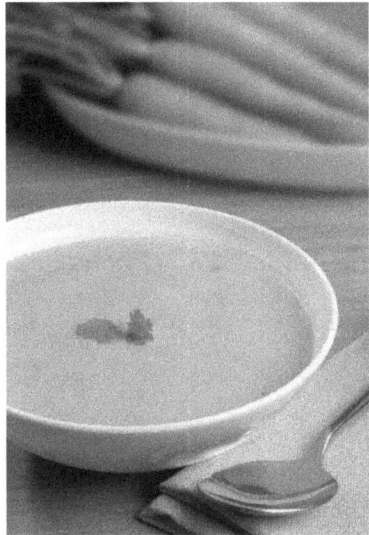

## 20 Awesome Raw Soups You Can't Live Without

RAW FOOD RECIPES FOR A HEALTHY LIFESTYLE

MEMBER OF THE RAW FOODS ASSOCIATION

BY KATHY TENNEFOSS

# RECIPES 4
## RAW FOOD

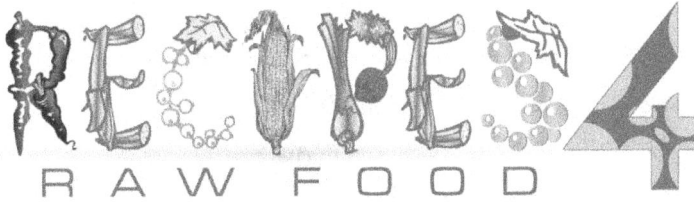

**20 Awesome Raw Soup Recipes You Can't Live Without**

**Sunny Cabana Publishing, L.L.C.**

**Fort Lauderdale, FL**

www.sunnycabanapublishing.com

By Kathy Tennefoss

All Rights Reserved © 2011 by Kathy Tennefoss

Published by Kathleen Tennefoss
Printed in the United States of America
Author: Kathy Tennefoss
Editor: Shawn M Tennefoss
13-digit ISBN: 9781936874064
10-digit ISBN: 1936874067
SECOND EDITION
Library of Congress Cataloging-in-Publication Data has been applied for

THIS BOOK IS DEDICATED TO MY DAD AND FRIEND JAMES KELLEY FOR PUSHING ME IN THE RIGHT DIRECTION ABOUT HEALTH FOOD AND LIVING A HEALTHY LIFE AND TO MY LOVING HUSBAND SHAWN TENNEFOSS FOR PUTTING UP WITH MY COMPUTER DIFFICULTIES AND TAKING THE TIME TO SHOW ME HOW TO PUT THIS TOGETHER ALONG WITH SHARING HIS LIFE AND JOURNEY WITH ME.

COVER DESIGN: KATHY & SHAWN TENNEFOSS

SECOND EDITION, 2011

ACKNOWLEDGEMENTS:

THANKS TO EVERYONE WHO ENCOURAGED AND INSPIRED ME AND GAVE ME GREAT IDEAS AND FEEDBACK IN THE RAW FOOD INDUSTRY, INCLUDING ONE OF MY MANY SISTERS HEATHER MCNERNEY, MY HUSBAND SHAWN M TENNEFOSS, MY DAD JAMES KELLEY, AND MELISSA HERNANDEZ AND HER WONDERFUL FAMILY! WITHOUT EVERYONE'S INPUT I WOULD NOT HAVE FINISHED THIS OR OTHER RAW FOOD RECIPE BOOKS THAT I HAVE IN THE WORKS! I AM EXTREMELY GRATEFUL TO EVERYONE!

IF YOU HAVE ANY SUGGESTIONS, COMMENTS, OR CORRECTIONS PLEASE FEEL FREE TO EMAIL ME AT recipes4rawfood@yahoo.com! I WOULD LOVE TO HEAR FROM YOU!

DISCLAIMER:

THE RESPONSIBILITY FOR ANY ADVERSE DETOXIFICATION EFFECTS RESULTING FROM USING THESE RECIPES DESCRIBED LIES NOT WITH THE AUTHOR OR DISTRIBUTORS OF THIS BOOK. THIS BOOK IS NOT INTENDED FOR MEDICAL ADVICE JUST AS SUGGESTION.

PLEASE ENJOY THESE RECIPES WITH YOUR FAMILIES!

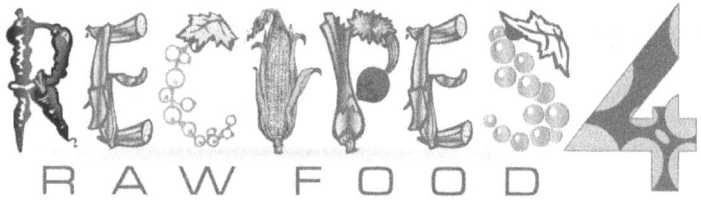

# RECIPES 4

## RAW FOOD

# 20 AWESOME RAW SOUPS YOU CAN'T LIVE WITHOUT

## RAW FOOD RECIPES FOR HEALTHY LIVING

### BY KATHY TENNEFOSS

# TABLE OF CONTENTS

IN THIS BOOK "20 AWESOME RAW SOUP RECIPES YOU CAN'T LIVE WITH-OUT" I HAVE GONE THROUGH ONLY SOME OF MY RECIPES THAT I FOUND ARE THE EASIEST TO MAKE WHEN YOU ARE SHORT ON TIME. EVERYONE IS BUSY BUT YOU STILL SHOULD MAKE THE TIME TO EAT A HEALTHY MEAL FOR YOU AND YOUR FAMILY. EATING HEALTHY IS ALSO ABOUT PUTTING FUN INTO YOUR MEALS BY INVOLVING THE WHOLE FAMILY AND HAVING THEM HELP AND GIVE THEIR INPUT SO THAT THEY FEEL LIKE THEY ARE CONTRIBUTING TO THEIR OWN HEALTH. WHEN YOUR CHILDREN GET OLDER THEY WILL REMEMBER THIS AND PASS THE HEALTHY LIVING ON TO THEIR FAMILY. I KNOW THIS FROM EXPERIENCE. I HAD A FATHER WHO ATE HEALTHY (MOSTLY VEGETARIAN MEALS) AND BIKED AND A MOTHER WHO ATE ONLY JUNK FOOD AND DID NOT EXERCISE WHATSOEVER. IT WAS A BATTLE AT OUR HOUSE OF WHAT TO EAT. I NEVER KNEW WHO TO GO WITH BUT AT LEAST I HAD THE OPTION AND THAT IS WHY I FEEL SO COMPELLED TO TELL OTHERS ABOUT HEALTHY EATING.

I DIDN'T REALIZE UNTIL I GOT OLDER HOW MY FATHER INFLUENCED ME AND MY FOOD CHOICES. MY MOTHER WAS ALWAYS SICK AND DID NOT TAKE CARE OF HERSELF VERY WELL AND THAT WAS TO HER DETRIMENT. I VOWED TO MYSELF AND

MY FAMILY THAT I WOULD TRY MY HARDEST TO SEEK OUT THE BEST QUALITY FOOD BY PURCHASING ORGANIC PRODUCE AND BY PREPARING THE FOOD AS TO NOT LOSE ITS NUTRITIONAL VALUE AND I HAVE STUCK TO THAT PROMISE FOR OVER 20 YEARS. I FEEL THAT THIS HAS HELPED ME AND MY FAMILY IMMENSELY AND I WANT TO PASS THE BENEFITS ON TO OTHERS SO THAT THEY TOO WILL FEEL THAT THEY ARE CONTRIBUTING TO A BETTER WAY OF LIFE!

PLEASE TRY ALL OF MY RECIPES AND PUT YOUR BEST FOOT FORWARD IN THE FIGHT FOR OBESITY, DIABETES, HEART DISEASE, CANCER, AND A SLEW OF OTHER AILMENTS THAT ARE FROM NOT EATING A HEALTHY DIET. ALSO REMEMBER THAT LIFE SHOULD BE FUN AND THAT EATING HEALTHY DOESN'T MEAN THAT YOU HAVE TO BE STRICT EVERY SINGLE DAY. IT'S THE SMALL EFFORTS THAT YOU PUT FORTH EVERYDAY THAT MAKE A DIFFERENCE IN THE LONG RUN! PEOPLE WILL START TO NOTICE YOUR HEALTHY GLOW AND HOW YOUNG YOU LOOK AND START TO ASK YOU HOW, WHAT, AND WILL YOU SHOW ME. THIS IS WHEN YOU WILL FEEL LIKE YOU HAVE MADE A DIFFERENCE IN THE WORLD.

# 20 Awesome Raw Soups That You Can't Live Without

www.Recipes4RawFood.com
By Kathy Tennefoss

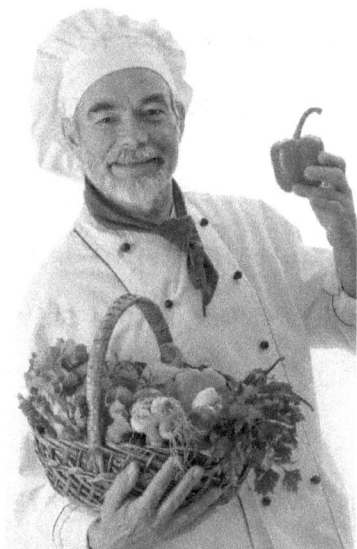

## Creamy Avocado and Cucumber Medley

4 Large Organic Cucumbers, peeled

4 Organic Celery Stalks

2 Hass Avocados peeled and pitted

2 Limes

4 Cups Purified Water

Put all the ingredients in the Vita-Mixer and chill and serve garnished with cilantro sprigs! Yum!

# Macho Gazpacho

4 Cups Roma Tomatoes

1 Cup diced and seeded Tomatoes

1 Cup peeled, seeded cucumber diced

2 Cup Red, Green, and Yellow Peppers

2 Limes squeezed into soup

2 Avocados cut into small pieces

3 Cloves of garlic crushed

1 Small bunch of Cilantro chopped

1 Small jalapeno, seeded and minced

1/2 Green onion minced

1 Teaspoon sea salt

Fresh Ground Black pepper

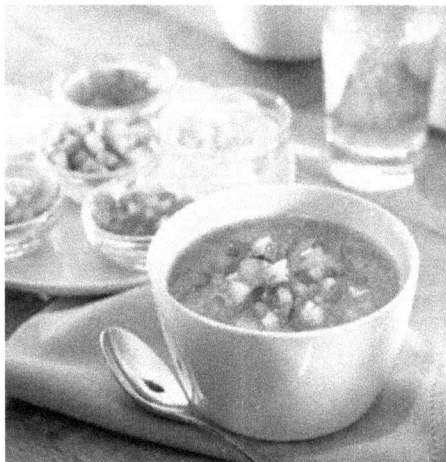


Puree the 4 cups of roma tomatoes and then add all the other ingredients and voila' you have Macho Gazpacho

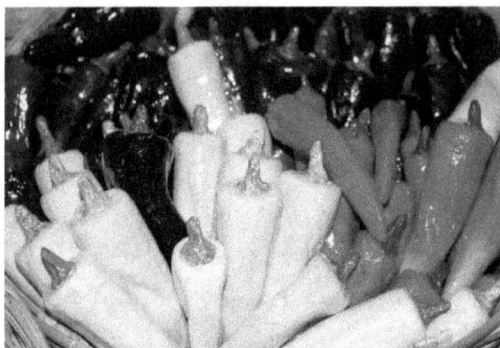

## CREAMY RED PEPPER SOUP

3 ORGANIC RED BELL PEPPERS SEEDED AND STEMS REMOVED

1 YOUNG COCONUT

2 CLOVES OF GARLIC

3 TABLESPOONS COLD PRESSED EXTRA VIRGIN OLIVE OIL

1 BUNCH OF ORGANIC CILANTRO

2 TEASPOONS OF SEA SALT

2 LIMES SQUEEZED

IF YOU LIKE IT SPICIER YOU CAN ADD A JALAPENO OR SOME CAYENNE PEPPER IT JUST DEPENDS ON HOW HOT YOU LIKE IT. USE ALL THE COCONUT MEAT AND JUICE. THEN MIX ALL THE INGREDIENTS IN A VITA-MIXER EXCEPT HALF OF THE CILANTRO (USE THE REST AS A GARNISH) AND YOU HAVE RED PEPPER SOUP. THIS IS A GREAT SOUP FOR BOOSTING YOUR VITAMIN C INTAKE SO EAT UP!

## CREAMY PEA SOUP

2 CUPS ORGANIC FRESH PEAS
2 CUPS OF PURIFIED WATER
1 LARGE RIPE AVOCADO
1 BUNCH BASIL LEAVES
3 CLOVES OF ORGANIC GARLIC
1 TEASPOON OF SEA SALT

BLEND ALL INGREDIENTS IN A VITA MIXER AND BLEND UNTIL SMOOTH!

## CREAMY CARROT FENNEL SOUP

4 CUPS OF PURIFIED WATER
4 ORGANIC CARROTS
1 LARGE AVOCADO
1 ORGANIC APPLE OF YOUR CHOICE
1 LARGE FENNEL BULB CHOPPED
1 TEASPOON OF SEA SALT
2 TABLESPOONS OF DILL WEED

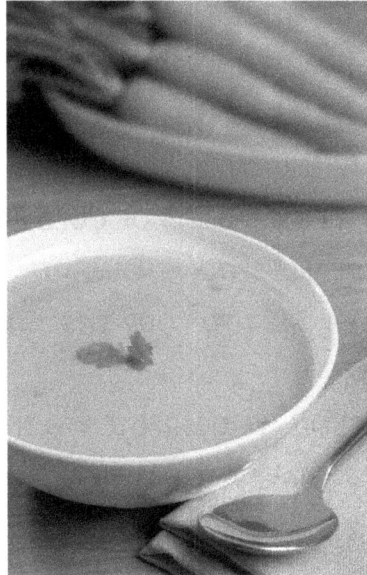

BLEND ALL INGREDIENTS IN A VITA-MIXER UNTIL CREAMY AND ENJOY!

# Thai Coconut Lemon grass Soup

2 Cups young
coconut meat
2 Cups coconut
water
3 Tablespoons of
Ginger
1 Tablespoon Thai
chili paste
2 Cloves of Garlic
1 Bunch of Organic Cilantro
2 Tablespoon of ground lemon grass
1/2 Bunch of Italian Parsley
3 Tablespoons of Cold Pressed Olive Oil
3 Tablespoons Tamari
Sea Salt to your tasting

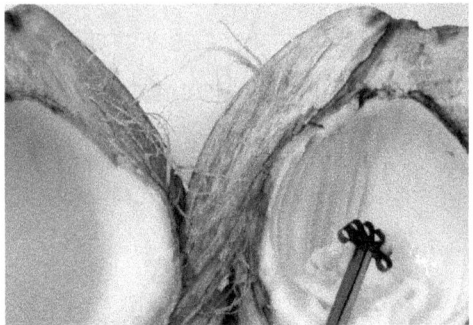

Blend all ingredients in the Vita-mixer and there
you have a great healthy meal!

# Spicy Watermelon Tomato Soup

4 Cups Watermelon seeded
2 cups any kind of Tomatoes
1 Cup Diced Tomatoes

1 Cup Diced Peeled Cucumber
1 Cup Diced Green and Red Peppers
1/4-1/2 (Depending on your tastes I like a lot of lime) Cup Key Lime Juice
1 Large Jalapeño Diced Into Small Pieces
1 Large Bunch of Cilantro chopped fine
1 Large Piece of Ginger peeled
Salt and Pepper to taste

First puree the 4 cups of watermelon and 2 cups of tomatoes along with the ginger in a Vita-Mixer. Then add all the other diced ingredients and eat up! This is great for summer or really anytime. It is very refreshing chilled!

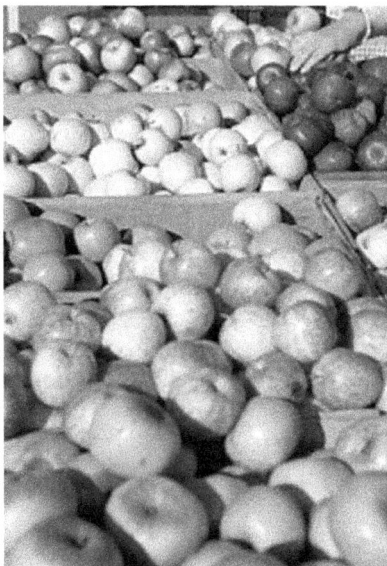

## Creamy Celery and Green Apple Soup

1 Bunch Organic Celery
4 Large Organic Granny Smith Apples
1/4 -1/2 Cup Lemon Juice (depends on your taste)
1/4 Cup Cold Pressed Olive Oil
2 Tablespoons of Coconut Butter (this you can find at most health food stores)
2 Cups Soaked Raw Macadamia nuts (soak for at

LEAST 2 HOURS)
1 CUP WATER OR TO YOUR THICKNESS
SEE SALT AND BLACK PEPPER TO TASTE
YOU CAN ADD CHOPPED PARSLEY FOR A GARNISH OR EVEN
BOTH RED AND GREEN APPLES MIXED TO GIVE IT A NICE
COLOR.

THIS IS A BIT OF A LABOR OF LOVE SOUP BUT IT IS VERY
TASTY! FIRST CUT THE CELERY INTO SMALL PIECES AND
ONLY 3 OF THE GRANNY SMITH APPLES AND PUT INTO THE
VITA MIXER.

ONCE THIS IS DONE DRAIN THE JUICE FROM THE PULP AND
SAVE BOTH. NOW WASH THE SOAKED MACADAMIA NUTS AND
THROW THEM IN THE VITA MIXER ALONG WITH THE
STRAINED JUICE, WATER, OLIVE OIL, LEMON JUICE, AND S &
P IF YOU WANT A THICKER SOUP YOU CAN ADD BACK SOME OF
THE PULP.
NOW THAT THIS IS DONE YOU GARNISH WITH THE LAST
GRANNY SMITH APPLE THAT YOU CUT INTO SMALL BITES SIZE
PIECES AND SERVE. YOU CAN ADD WHITE TRUFFLE OIL FOR
AN EVEN RICHER SOUP OR IF YOU ARE HAVING QUESTS DUE
TO THE PRICE OF THE OIL.

# Raw Creamy Celery Soup

1 Bunch of celery
1/2 Cup Olive Oil
1/4 Cup Lemon Juice
4 Cups of Water
2 Teaspoons of Agave nectar
1 Cup soaked Raw Cashews
3/4 Cup of Parsley

You can also top this soup off with chopped avocado, sliced carrots, or chopped red pepper and parsley.

Blend all ingredients in a Vita mixer until smooth and creamy. If you want the soup thicker just use 1 cup less water in the recipe. This is great soup for the summer chilled or right out of the Vita mixer!

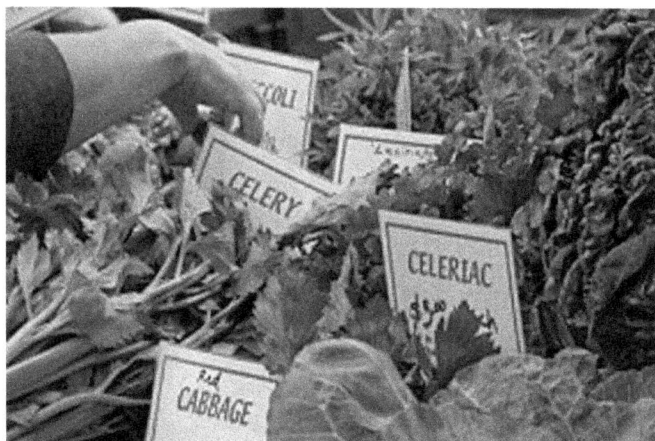

# Raw Tomato Soup

8 Large Tomatoes

2 Cloves of Garlic peeled

$\frac{1}{4}$ Cup of Lime Juice

1/8 Cup of Olive Oil

Salt and Pepper to your liking

Tablespoon of Chopped Basil

Tablespoon of Chopped Oregano

This is one of the easiest raw soups to make! Just blend all ingredients with a Vita mixer until smooth consistency and garnish with a few basil sprigs!

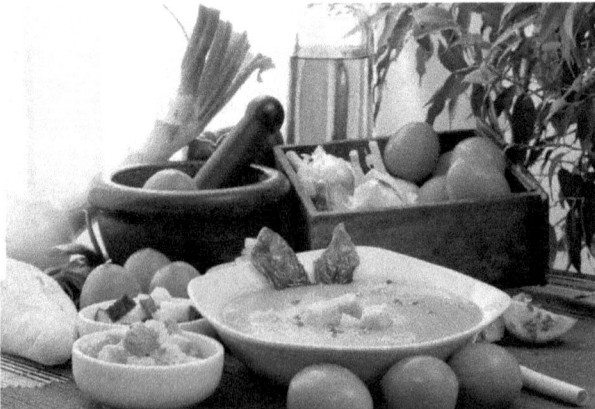

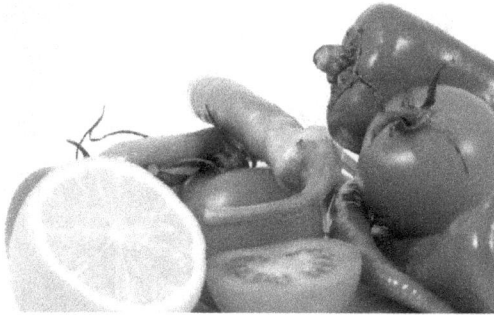

# Tomato and Poblano Chili Soup (this is a hot one)

1 Cup of sun dried tomatoes Soaked for 4-5 hours

2-3 Dried Poblanos soaked for 4-5 hours

3 Cups of Water

½ Cup of Lemon Juice

¼ Cup of Olive Oil

1 small peeled cucumber

Chopped Parsley

Chopped Cilantro

Salt and Pepper to taste

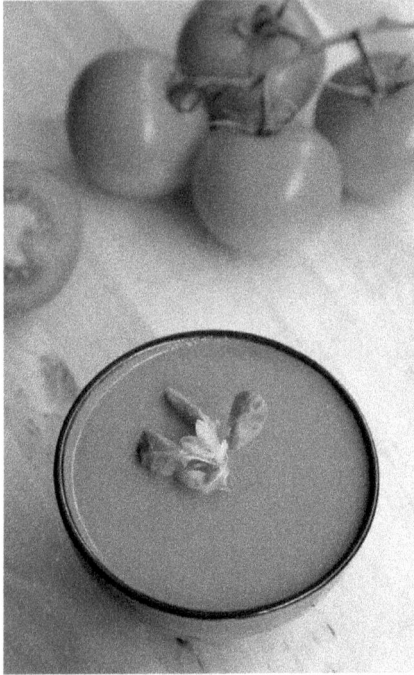

Rinse the soaked tomatoes and poblano chilies and put them along with the rest of the ingredients in the Vita mixer and garnish with Cilantro and extra slice of lemons or limes!

# CREAMY BUTTERNUT SQUASH SOUP

3 Cups peeled and cut into smaller pieces for the Vita Mixer

1/8 Cup Olive Oil

1/8 Cup of Raw Peanut Butter

2 Tablespoons of Parsley

1 teaspoon of Curry powder

$\frac{1}{4}$ Lime Juice

$\frac{3}{4}$ Cup of Water

Sea Salt of Braggs to your liking

1 Tablespoon of agave nectar

Mix all of the above ingredients into a Vita Mixer until smooth and garnish with fresh parsley sprigs!

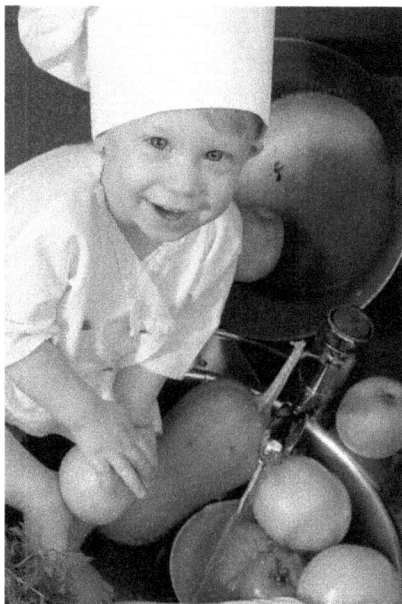

# SPINACH SOUP

- 1 CUP OF ALMOND MILK
- 1 CUP OF WATER
- 5 CUPS OF SPINACH
- 2 SMALL CUCUMBERS PEELED
- 1 CLOVE OF GARLIC
- $\frac{1}{4}$ CUP OF ALMOND BUTTER
- 1/8 CUP OF LIME JUICE
- 1/8 CUP OF HEMP OIL
- SALT AND PEPPER TO TASTE OR BRAGGS IF YOU LIKE

MIX ALL INGREDIENTS IN THE VITA MIXER AND GARNISH WITH A FEW SLICES OF CUCUMBER!

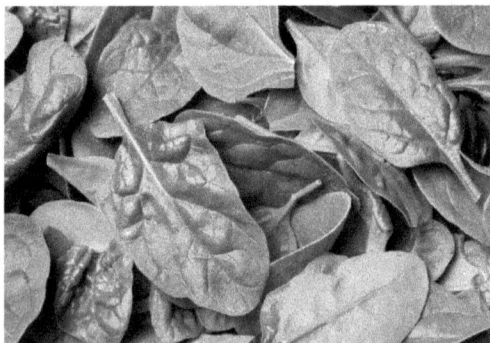

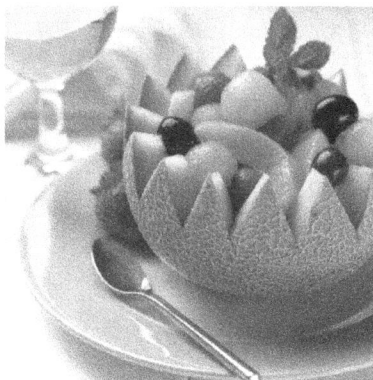

## SWEET SUMMER WATERMELON SOUP

6 CUPS OF WATERMELON

1 CUP HONEY DEW MELLON

1 CUP OF ICE

$\frac{1}{2}$ CUP OF PINEAPPLE JUICE

CHOPPED MINT

MIX ALL INGREDIENTS IN A VITA MIXER EXCEPT 1 CUP OF THE WATERMELON (CUT INTO SMALL CHUNKS AND USE AS A GARNISH)! THIS IS A GREAT SOUP TO COOL YOU OFF IN THE SUMMER!

## MANGO MADNESS

4 LARGE RIPE MANGOES PEELED AND CUT INTO PIECES
(JUST SO THAT THE MANGO FLESH IS SEPARATED
FROM THE SEED)
$\frac{1}{4}$ CUP LIME JUICE
2 CUP ORANGE JUICE
3 PITTED DATES
CHOPPED MINT

MIX ALL INGREDIENTS EXCEPT ONE OF THE MANGOES
(SAVE IT FOR GARNISH IN THE SOUP) IN A VITA
MIXER AND GARNISH WITH THE EXTRA MANGO AND
CHOPPED MINT!

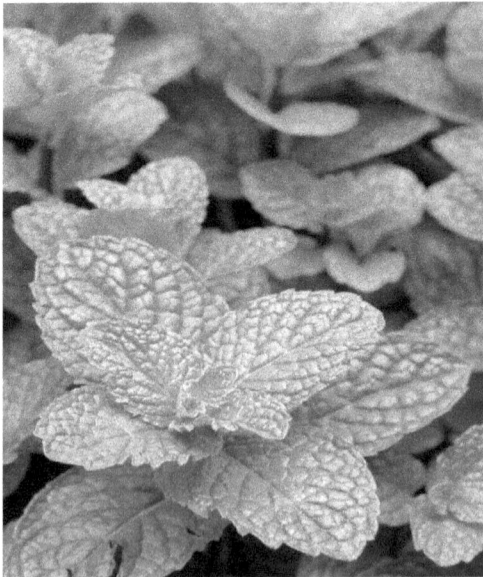

# PEANUT SOUP

2 CUPS WATER

1 CUP ORANGE JUICE

2 RIPE BANANAS

1 TEASPOON CURRY POWDER

1 CUP NATURAL PEANUT BUTTER

$\frac{1}{4}$ CUP LIME JUICE

1 TABLESPOON PEELED GINGER ROOT

1 CLOVE OF GARLIC

CHOPPED CILANTRO

MIX ALL INGREDIENTS EXCEPT THE CILANTRO IN A VITA MIXER AND BLEND UNTIL SMOOTH. GARNISH WITH CHOPPED PEANUTS AND CHOPPED CILANTRO! YUM!

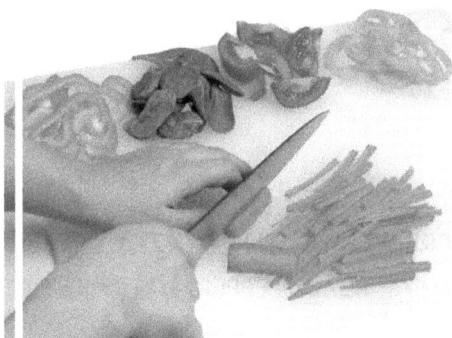

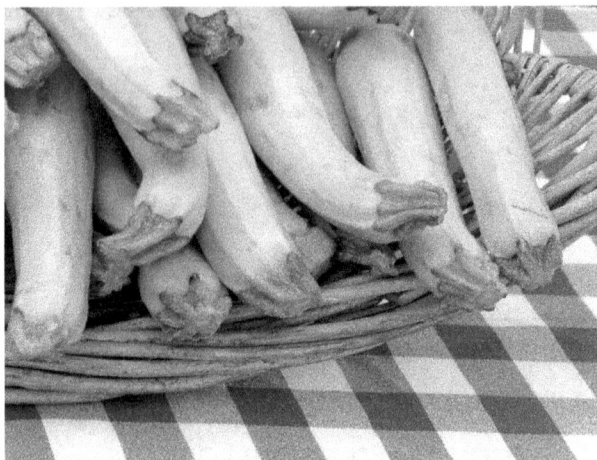

## Black Pepper and Zucchini Soup

4 Peeled Zucchinis

4 Stalks of Celery

2 Cups of water

$\frac{1}{4}$ cup of olive oil

1 Tablespoon of Black Pepper

1 Clove of Garlic

Salt to taste

Blend all ingredients in a vita mixer and garnish with more black pepper! Spicy but good!

# Coconut and Macadamia Nut soup

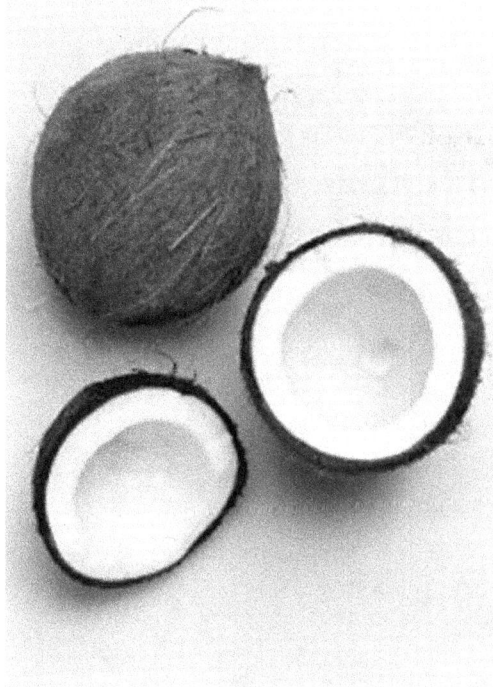

2 Cups Raw Macadamia Nuts soaked for several hours

1 raw coconut Scooped and the water saved

2 cups extra coconut water

$\frac{1}{4}$ lime juice

1/8 cup of Macadamia nut oil

Salt and Pepper to taste

Cilantro for garnish

Drain the soaked macadamia nuts and put the rest of the ingredients in the Vita mixer and blend until smooth. Garnish with chopped macadamia nuts, raw shredded coconut, and cilantro! Yum you will have more friends than you want with this soup!

## Summer Romaine Soup

- 1 Head of romaine lettuce
- 2 stalks of celery
- 1 small peeled cucumber
- 1 cup of water
- $\frac{1}{4}$ cup lemon juice
- 1 small piece of ginger peeled
- Salt and pepper to taste
- Garnish with chopped cilantro

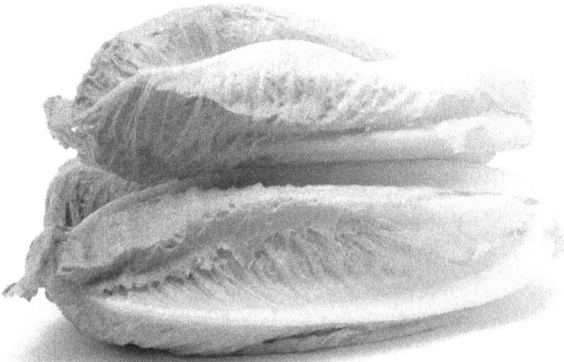

Blend all ingredients in a vita mixer and blend until smooth. Garnish with chopped cilantro! This is a nice a refreshing summer soup!

# Kale Nutrition Soup

6 Cups of Kale
2 cups of water
1 peeled cucumber
$\frac{1}{4}$ cup of lemon juice
1/8 cup of olive oil
$\frac{1}{2}$ cup of flat leaf parsley
3 celery stalks
Salt and pepper to taste

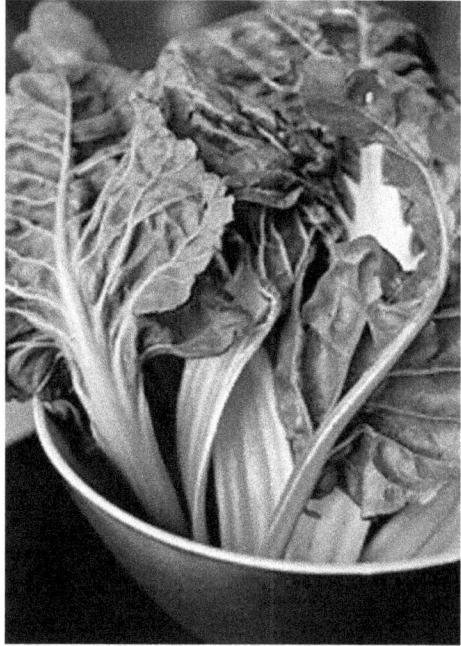

Mix all ingredients together in a Vita Mixer and blend until smooth. The consistency will be a little on the thicker side and garnish with chopped cucumbers! This is delish and nutrish!

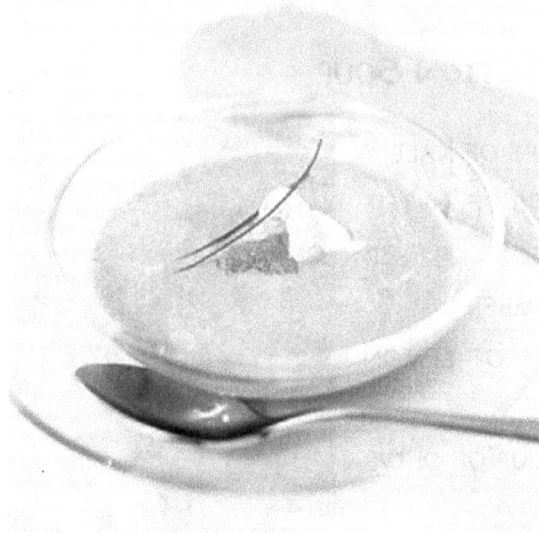

I HOPE YOU ENJOY THIS BOOK ON RAW SOUP RECIPES! I WANT TO HELP OTHERS ON THEIR JOURNEY TO BETTER HEALTH.

**IF YOU ARE NOT SURE ABOUT HOW TO USE A RAW YOUNG COCONUT HERE IS AN EASY SOLUTION FOR YOU.**

Young coconuts are not just a wonderful delicacy. There are so many ways in which young coconuts do wonders for our health like lowering cholesterol, reduce the risk of heart disease, and has anti-inflammatory benefits for the body.

In the tropical region it is considered to be the most important fruit, simply because people know of its medicinal properties and also because of its mineral rich water, such as potassium, copper, iron, calcium, ascorbic acid, and B-complex vitamins. Young coconuts are highly nutritious in nature and have medicative qualities, which are very good for your heart, liver and kidneys. In fact, the latest research reports suggest that apart from its nutritional features the young coconuts are reported to reduce the viral load of Human Immuno-deficiency Virus or HIV.

It's also known for its natural electrolyte source. Also, it is believed that many people living in third world countries have actually been saved by these young coconuts. The coconuts in their young age happen to be the most health enhancing. Not to mention the fact that it's similar to blood plasma and has been used in emergency blood transfusions.

These are just few of the benefits of young coconuts. Now let's discuss how to open and eat a young coconut as many people find this a tough job to do:

The best and simplest way to open a coconut is to put the coconut inside a plastic bag, tie its ends and just swing it on any flat, hard surface, which would shatter the young coconut into shards. You can get the meat simply by separating coconut meat from the husk in this fashion. Use the plastic bag to retain the coconut water. Now hold the plastic bag so that the liquid settles down at the bottom. You can now puncture a hole and get a glassful of coconut juice. It's as easy as 1, 2, 3. .

The meats of young coconut are quite soft and can be scooped out with a spoon or a knife. However, the suggested way is to use a small knife with a flexible blade, which would allow it to follow the contour of the shell while undercutting the meat out of the shell.

The young coconuts are great choice for the summers as they quite easy to prepare and they are available at most grocery store. Young coconuts are a great enhancer to various drinks, especially tropical drinks, smoothies, pies, and dinner dishes as well. Humid countries rely heavily on coconut-based foods.

ABOUT THE AUTHOR:

B.S. Science in Physical Anthropology minor in business, and Culinary Arts Degree. Advocate for organic, vegetarian, vegan, raw food diets, writing, yoga, swimming, biking, and running 5 K's! I have been a vegetarian/vegan/raw foodist for over 20 years. I have also worked in real estate for over ten years and have several websites to help people who are interested in raw food http://www.Recipes4RawFood.com and http://www.RawFoodForToday.com . I have also started the Raw Foods Association with my husband so that others can become members of a larger healthy group and its website is www.RawFoodsAssociation.com!

For more information on how to order books, original articles, become a member of the Raw Foods Association, and updates on future projects go to www.rawfoodfortoday.com or www.recipes4rawfood.com!

Please feel free to email me with suggestions, comments, or corrections at recipes4rawfood@yahoo.com.

Recipes 4 Raw Food

1314 E Las Olas Blvd

Fort Lauderdale, FL 33301

www.ingramcontent.com/pod-product-compliance
Lightning Source LLC
Chambersburg PA
CBHW060706280326
41933CB00012B/2318